Healthily & Holistically

Transition to

Working Motherhood

A Gentle, Practical Guide to Returning
to Work After Having a Baby

Table of Contents

Preface **8**

How to use this book **9**

   It wasn't simple. 9

   What this book is not: 10

   How to use this book 11

Prenatal **12**

   Activity: 13

   Emotional 15

   Visualization: 16

   Sources of emotional support 16

  Sleep 17

   Body attunement scan 18

  Nutrition 18

   Journal prompt: 19

   Tips: 20

Financial..20

    "Use what you have" – Effectively accessing financial resources..................20

    Financial Reframe..21

Childcare 22

    Prompt: 22

    Inform yourself: 22

Social 24

    Relationship audit.. 24

    Exercise: 25

    Journal prompts – accepting help 26

    "No thanks."..28

    "Party of two?" 28

Physical..29

    Coloring page...29

    Journal prompt:..30

    Bodies at work... 32

Postpartum 34

Emotional...35

    What to expect with baby blues..35

    Journal prompt:..36

Sleep 38

    Coloring page...38

    Making the bedroom a sanctuary 39

    Sleep hygiene:.. 39

    Mantras for rest...40

Nutrition 40

    Support yourself and ask for support. 41

Financial 42

    Money worries 42

    "Hit the snooze button" 42

    "Don't mind if I do..." 42

Childcare 42

    Prompt: 43

    Communication: 43

Social 44

    Prompt 44

    Social scripts 44

    Gratitude 45

Physical 45

    Gratitude 45

    Post-partum movement tips: 46

Pre TransitionBack to Work **48**

Emotional 49

    Yellow flags: 50

Sleep 50

    Planning for sleep transition 50

    Sleep beliefs 51

Nutrition 51

    Things to think about - family meals. 51

    Things to think about - daytime meals 52

    Things to think about - baby 53

    Reframe 53

Financial 53

    Audit 53

Childcare 54
    Things to consider: 55
Social 56
    Audit: Cup-fillers and cup-drainers 56
    Connecting with important figures 56
Physical 57
    Journal prompt: 57
    Audit: 58
    Reframe 58

Early Back to Work **60**
Emotional 61
    "My best is enough." 62
    Thoughts-feelings-behavior 62
Sleep 63
    "Partner renegotiation" 63
    "Sleepy affirmations" 65
    Strategies for the sleepless night 66
    Tips for the next day 66
Nutrition 67
    Audit 67
    What's your food-mood relationship? 68
Financial 70
Childcare 71
    Design your routine 72
Social 72
    Prompt: Nurturing old relationships 73
    Opening new doors 75

Physical 75

You could: 76

Settling In **78**

Emotional 79

"What is your why?" 79

Journal prompt 80

Sleep 80

Audit: 80

Nutrition 81

Audit: 81

Action: 81

Financial 82

Childcare 83

Audit: Is your childcare balanced? 83

Social 83

Audit: 83

Physical 84

"My body, my why." 85

Journal prompt 85

Final thoughts **87**

Preface

How to use this book

The transition back to work after childbirth is often an invisible transition. So overshadowed by the seismic shift of welcoming a new baby into the world, the return to work can come as an afterthought – for the new mother and for the people in her orbit.

This workbook is meant to provide space for the spaceless expectation to "just" go back to work. My goal is to offer reflections, exercises, and activities to help support new mothers in gently transitioning and tending to their wellness so the return is not so bumpy.

The publishing industry doesn't have much to say on this topic. When I identified that gap, I sat down to write *Employed Motherhood: Healthily and Holistically Transition Back to Work after Having a Baby.* This is a companion piece where I translate some of those insights into tangible activities.

It wasn't simple.

There are so many moving parts to working motherhood; it can be hard to know where to start, what to prioritize, and how deep to dive into certain areas. To that end, I want to acknowledge this workbook does not strive to say it all.

I chose to organize the book into sections corresponding to the major periods of transition, starting from the prenatal period to the immediate post-partum period, the preparation for return to work, and a final "settling in" section. Because maternity leaves vary in length, I tried to avoid specifics about what age a baby might be in preparation for returning to work and settling in. For some moms with just the briefest of leaves (I see you!), the immediate post-partum period is the preparation for return to work, so exercises in either section might apply.

I've broken down each section into the major areas of challenge I've identified both personally and professionally, including through eight in-depth interviews I conducted as part of my research for the *Employed Motherhood* book. Each section starts with a focus on emotions since that's the core of my practice. From there (in no particular order), I include activities on sleep, nutrition, finance, childcare, relationships, and physical wellness. Each of these topics deserves its own library of material; I've boiled it down to a few key elements of focus to set you up for success.

Throughout the book, you'll see a variety of activities, including free-form journaling, brainstorming, and coloring, as well as mindfulness exercises and exercises inspired by cognitive behavioral therapy.

What this book is not:

There are so many things I can't hope to accomplish here. This is by no means an exhaustive list, but by way of acknowledgment:

I couldn't hope to talk about where you'll be in a year. There's so much to cover perinatally that it wasn't realistic to stretch too far into the future. You may be making major career moves, revisiting your industry, or your relationship to work in general. You may be continuing to grow your family.

Speaking of families, this book doesn't focus on the rich, complex universe that is sibling dynamics. Whether you have older children already, are expecting again, or are in the family-planning mode, everything changes as you add more tiny humans to the mix. Considering the number of variables already in play, it didn't make sense for me to try to play four-dimensional chess. I know that there are excellent coaches and resources out there that specialize in sibling dynamics and parenting multiples.

In terms of relationships, while I occasionally refer to a partner, this is a book for moms – partnered or not. Some of the activities can be completed as a couple's exercise, but my primary focus is on you and helping you get clear on your needs and wants. I also want this book to be inclusive of different kinds of families – two-mom families (including the non-birthing partner), families that formed out of surrogacy or adoption, so please feel free to skip any sections that don't apply (for example, ones that refer to physical recovery from childbirth, if you are the non-birthing partner).

On the work front, this is not a legal handbook. A not-small number of mothers will need legal advice and protections when returning to work (and oh, I do see you!), but there are too many contexts across readership for me to dip my toe in these murky waters. Legal counsel (pro-bono or paid), HR offices, union offices, trusted colleagues, mentors, and others may all be resources for you if you find yourself in need.

This is not a book about office dynamics. There will be mentions of coworkers and how to handle certain situations, but that's also too rich a vein for me to tap into fully.

Crucially, although this book talks about perinatal mood disorders, this is not a psychiatric guide. If you think you might have a mood disorder, please see a trusted medical professional.

How to use this book

Start where you are. Skip around. Use what resonates – and if you love a certain exercise, check the addendum for additional pages to continue your line of thought.

If you want to involve a partner, I recommend doing exercises individually and then comparing them whenever you have a quiet moment. I highly recommend doing this book in parallel with another working mom to structure a conversation and help facilitate creative juices.

I want this book to be a starting point for many conversations. I hope it gives you ideas and serves as an invitation to include other people, including professionals, into your journey: an OB, a nutritionist, a coach, a therapist, and a fellow working mom who has been through the trenches.

Whatever this book is for, I hope it is part of a gentle, relaxing, self-care practice. Even if it becomes a small corner of your hectic life, know that you're doing something valuable for yourself and your baby.

Prenatal

When you first learn you're going to become a parent, a countdown clock might start in your mind. So much to do, so little time. I want to validate that feeling. Yes, it's true: your to-do list just got a lot longer. And yes, many of those tasks need to be done soon before that "deadline" comes screaming into the world, but not everything.

This is my invitation to you to practice setting – and respecting – priorities. There are only 24 hours in a day, and some of them will have to be used for sleeping. Don't worry; the important things will get done. Everything else can just wait.

Activity:

Use this space to brainstorm your priorities for this prenatal period. What is top of mind? What's the "small stuff" that maybe you can try not to sweat? Make a list, doodle, whatever feels good. Research shows that getting tasks out of your head and onto paper helps eliminate those nagging doubts that sometimes get in the way of a good night's sleep.

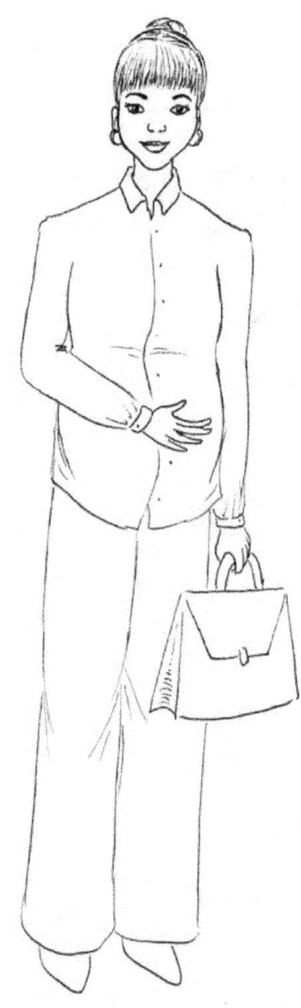

Emotional

Whatever thoughts and feelings are swirling around your head about your pregnancy, your upcoming leave, and all the life changes – upcoming and already in progress – this workbook is here to offer you tools and opportunities to validate them, reflect on them, and let go of the ones that are not working for you.

One way we can do this is through a 'reframing' exercise – taking negative thoughts and then considering them in a positive light.

Consider an area currently stressing you: discussing leave with your team, looking for childcare, physical challenges – anything that is top of mind right now. Set a timer for five minutes and let yourself pour it all out onto the page.

After the five minutes, list the five most powerful statements in the left-hand column below, and reflect on a positive reframe that you can put in the right-hand column opposite.

Once you complete the table, give yourself another five minutes to rewrite your story in a positive light. When negative thoughts resurface on this topic, use this page as a support to help you redirect back to the reframe.

(Repeat, with new topics, as needed!)

Example: Taking leave

Negative Thoughts	Positive Reframe
I'm going to miss out on so much at work.	I'm about to transform and will bring back a better self when I return.
My absence will add extra stress to everyone else.	I deserve this time off for me and my family.

Negative Brain Dump:

____

____

____

____

____

Positive Revision:

Visualization:

Another way to nudge our brain away from negative storytelling is to commit to envisioning an ideal situation. Rather than worrying about the logistics of your leave, spend time visualizing other things, like what you want to return to. When you focus on the outcome, your brain will be more receptive to creating and recognizing solutions.

Sources of emotional support

There's no escaping stress altogether during this major life transition, but it is important to manage it wherever possible. Most pregnant women experience disruption to their sleep, which also increases their risk factors for perinatal mood and anxiety disorders, also known as PMADs. Post-partum Support International is a resource-saturated organization to support those experiencing PMADs, encompassing support groups, peer support, provider directories, and even a helpline.

What other sources of support do you have? What are other local or online resources you might tap into?

1. ____

2. ____

3. ____

Sleep

Nap guilt is real. I hear it all the time from expecting and new moms. It can feel overwhelming to have so much to do at work, at home, and in your personal life. Who has time for a nap?

Give yourself permission to rest. Labor is – as the name describes – work. You may be experiencing insomnia or multiple wake-ups during the night, courtesy of your bladder. You may have another child who doesn't always sleep through the night or a partner who snores. You may feel pressure to grind through all your projects because you've got the birth deadline coming up. Consider resting as a gift to yourself and your baby.

As your due date arrives and you're setting up post-partum leave, consider taking some time off beforehand to build in a period of rest. Regardless of how you arrange your work schedule, let yourself nap when possible.

Prompt: What are your current beliefs around rest? How can you transform those beliefs, if needed, to better meet this season?

____

____

____

____

____

____

____

Body attunement scan

Do this alone or with your little one as part of a feeding or nap (if it feels good!)

Start by lying on your back, arms at your side, palms facing up, and legs extended. Begin at your toes and concentrate your awareness on each part of your body, slowly and intentionally. Move upwards through every part of your body, taking time to note any sensations, feelings, or insights that come up with each one. If a certain area generates more intense feelings, there is no need for judgment. You can simply breathe into those feelings for as long as it feels good before moving on to the next.

If you would like to journal about any part of the attunement experience, leave some notes here:

____

____

____

____

____

____

Nutrition

Nourishing baby:

Bottle or breast? There are more than just two options for feeding your baby. In addition to exclusive formula feeding and exclusive breastfeeding, some families incorporate multiple options.

- Pumping - you can feed your baby breast milk from a bottle, exclusively or as needed (for scheduling reasons, latching challenges, or to incorporate other caregivers in feeding)

- Formula and breast milk - depending on your milk supply, baby's weight gain, and other needs and requirements, you may want to incorporate both formula and breast milk.

You might not know which of the many choices is going to work for you and your baby until after the birth. (And things can change, week to week!) For now, educate yourself on the different methods.

> **LACTATION ISSUES**
>
> - Blocked Duets
> - Dysphoric Milk Ejection Reflex (D-MER)
> - Mastitis
> - Milk Blister

Nourishing yourself:

Our attitudes about food can inform the beliefs that we pass on to our children. Take time to reflect on your beliefs around nutrition to see how you can take a deliberate, intentional approach to nourishing both yourself and your baby.

Journal prompt:

As you think about your goals for feeding your baby, ask yourself, "What are my beliefs around feeding myself? To dig deeper into that question, ask yourself:

Where did those beliefs come from? Why do I make certain food choices? How would I describe my relationship to food?"

> **Tips:**
>
> - Stock the fridge and pantry with healthy foods and snacks.
>
> - Cook a little extra of your favorite soups, stews, and freezer meals, and store them.
>
> - Consider organizing a meal train for after your due date – or, if you have sufficient support during your post-partum period, schedule it for your return to work.
>
> - Investigate local meal delivery services.
>
> - If friends and family offer favors, think about how they can facilitate your shopping and cooking.

Financial

A lot is coming down the pipeline, from increased medical bills, childcare costs, and infinite piles of baby gear. Consider using this time to get some ducks in a row around health insurance, tax credits, and parental leave – paid and unpaid. In most cases, there's time after birth to investigate these things more deeply, so there's no rush.

Get what you can off your plate now, and don't worry about the rest until later.

"Use what you have" – Effectively accessing financial resources.

- Check your health insurance: Many insurers offer new moms a free breast pump or other resources.

- Check your FMLA status at work and any red tape around accessing it. (This might be time-sensitive – in some cases, you have a deadline for notifying your employer after the birth.)

- Ask your employer / HR department about the benefits available for families (Dependent daycare assistance, family medical insurance), family leave policies, and the ability to extend your paid leave period with unpaid leave or part-time work. Have your partner do the same.

- If you or your partner are self-employed, ask your CPA/bookkeeper how your added dependents might change your tax burden.

- If you have a family budget, incorporate a placeholder number for childcare based on the local market.

- Inform yourself about local second-hand stores or buy-nothing groups that can help provide affordable or free resources. You may have mom-friends and relatives who are ready to pass along hand-me-downs, such as clothes, strollers, and toys (If accepting a used car seat, check its expiration date – yes, car seats expire as their plastic degrades – and be sure it comes from a trusted source who can vouch that it has been in no accidents.)

- Put some bills on autopay to save bandwidth later.

Financial Reframe

Take some time to complete this exercise yourself. If you have a partner, you could also ask them to do it independently and then compare your answers, making sure to let each person speak uninterrupted for an equal amount of time before moving into a discussion.

1. What are your thoughts, feelings, and concerns about money as it relates to parenthood that are no longer serving you?

____

____

____

2. What are the sources of those beliefs?

____

____

____

3. How can you reframe your beliefs around money to better serve you in this transitional period?

____

____

____

For partners: Where do your attitudes towards money converge? Where do they differ? Where can you start to move towards common ground?

____

____

____

Childcare

Tell someone you're expecting, and chances are, within a few minutes, they'll ask you, "So, what are you going to do about childcare?" There are so many options, so before you commit to any specific situation, take some time to think about your ideal setup – then inform yourself about what's available in your area and see how the two line up.

Remember, while you may have a vision of what you want right now, you still haven't met your baby and experienced their temperament. Babies are wonderfully adaptable, but it may turn out your social butterfly would flourish in a group setting, or you may have a baby who strongly prefers one-on-one interactions. You won't know until you meet them, so stay flexible where possible.

Prompt:

- What's your ideal childcare situation? What kind of setting is your child in (Your home, another home, or a center)? What kind of caregivers do they have (Family, friends, a nanny, an international au pair, a daycare provider, you and/or your partner)? What other children, if any, are present? How much time per day are they receiving care?

  - If you have any non-negotiables (specific hours, etc.), list them here.

1. ____

2. ____

3. ____

Inform yourself:

- What's available in your area? What do other people in your profession do? Try to get insight from a range of people, including online local parenting groups, neighbors, and friends – but take what you hear with a grain of salt. Sometimes, people love to share horror stories. Don't forget, just because your perfect childcare setup doesn't exist in your area doesn't mean you can't create something that's right for you.

____

____

____

- What's the best thing about your childcare situation?

____

____

____

- What's the biggest challenge?

____

____

____

- What do you wish you knew before you had your baby?

____

____

____

After speaking with a variety of people, which insights do you find most helpful? What options do you want to explore further?

- If you're in an area with high demand for childcare, you may need to put your name on a waiting list for popular centers or enter into an agreement with a nanny. Take a deep breath, find out if there's a non-refundable deposit, and do your best.

  - For a daycare, consider things like hours of operation, sick/COVID-19 policy, nap schedules, communication practices, breast milk and formula policies, indoor/outdoor time, and screen time.

  - For a nanny: hourly schedule, sick policy, vaccines, driving record, references, vacation/PTO, and communication.

  - For a nanny share, ask the other families about the location, payment arrangements, behavior policies, and communication (and the nanny questions above).

Social

"Working mom's web of support."

In this time when change might seem like the only constant, take a moment to think about where you are in terms of your relationships – old and new, steady and variable, and intimate and professional.

Some relationships that might serve you include:

- Professionals: There are so many kinds of professionals trained to provide support during the pre- and post-natal period. Sometimes, they provide one-on-one support; other times, they might be the gateway to a community. Many are in-person services; others are available online. A lot of these practitioners are self-employed, local business owners (fellow working mamas!), so supporting them is a win-win.

  - Doula (pre- or post-partum) - many offer birthing classes.

  - Health professionals: the pediatrician, lactation consultant, and obstetrician (also may offer birthing classes).

  - Mental health professionals such as perinatal mental health professionals, also known as PMH-C's.

  - Wellness professionals: massage therapists, personal trainers, acupuncturists, and yoga instructors.

- Mentors: formal or informal, finding other people who have already lived the experience. You might find these mentors in your current workplace or broader professional network, in your family or friend group. There may be other working moms in your local community or online. Don't underestimate the value of having a safe relationship to vent your fears and pick up tips.

- Social network:

  - Local mom groups such as stroller strides.

  - Online forums, 'online dating for moms.'

Relationship audit

Even longstanding relationships can benefit from a renewal in this period. As you enter working motherhood, you likely will shuffle your priorities. Even if your values stay the same, the new perspective and daily experiences may make you see things – and people – in a different way.

It's normal for friendships to evolve during this season. You may find yourself gravitating towards other moms – or struggling to relate to moms who have dramatically different parenting approaches. (Before childbirth, who knew napping could be such a hot-button issue?) Sometimes, these changes prove to be permanent, a new phase in your life. But it may just be a temporary season: certain relationships take the backburner during these intensive parenting years while others come to the foreground. Please take a moment to reflect on where your relationships stand now and what you hope for them in the future. Be intentional and deliberate, but recognize these feelings might well shift.

If you have a partner – even if you've been coupled up for a long time – the birth of a child represents a new phase in your relationship. You may need to shift your responsibilities dramatically during the prenatal period, and it's never too early to start discussing what you expect that relationship to look like. Will you divide and conquer? Is your partner taking tasks off your plate?

Exercise:

Building the web – Where's the gap?

Think about your current relationships and reflect: What support do you have currently?

Then, looking at that reflection and the list above, ask yourself: What support do you anticipate needing? Where can you find it?

Here's a small example to think about: In your first 1-2 weeks post-partum, you will likely have out-of-the-house medical appointments for you and or your baby. Who will accompany you? If the answer isn't immediately obvious, reflect on whom you could ask for assistance and how you might phrase the request.

Journal prompts – accepting help

"I can do it myself." Is this your mantra? If so, you're not alone. For many working moms, doing things on your own is a deeply ingrained pattern. When it comes to asking for help, the juice isn't always worth the squeeze. But nobody parents alone. Think about getting yourself into a mindset to be able to accept support.

What would it take to say 'yes' when support is offered?

What would it take to be able to ask for help?

To whom would you feel most comfortable asking for help? From whom would you feel most comfortable accepting help? Why?

Building a resilient web takes time. What steps can you take today to start to build yours?

"No thanks."

The world is full of people ready to offer unsolicited comments, advice, and opinions, but somehow, during pregnancy, they seem to surface in record numbers. Relatives, colleagues, friends, and even total strangers may take it upon themselves to give you their two cents on parenting, childbirth, and issues big and small. What you're eating, wearing, drinking, buying, how much you're exercising, the weight you're gaining or not gaining – it seems like everything is up for grabs.

"Party of two?"

One of the biggest decisions a mom makes in the prenatal period is who they want to have with them for the birth. The first factor to consider is any rules put in place by the hospital or birth center where you plan to deliver. Within those constraints, this is the time to think about who you want in the room with you: a partner, another family member, a doula, support for the partner, or a close friend.

In this decision-making process, you take center stage. Think about your non-negotiables – then discuss with your partner, if you have one, to see if they have anything to add. Do they want a support person? Do you have any thoughts about who that might be and what role they can have in the birth?

Now's a good time to think about who you want to visit (or if you prefer no visits at all) – at the hospital, in the early post-partum period – and to communicate that with your circles. Put a few planned responses in your pocket in case of some unexpected visitors or untimely requests.

Physical

Coloring page

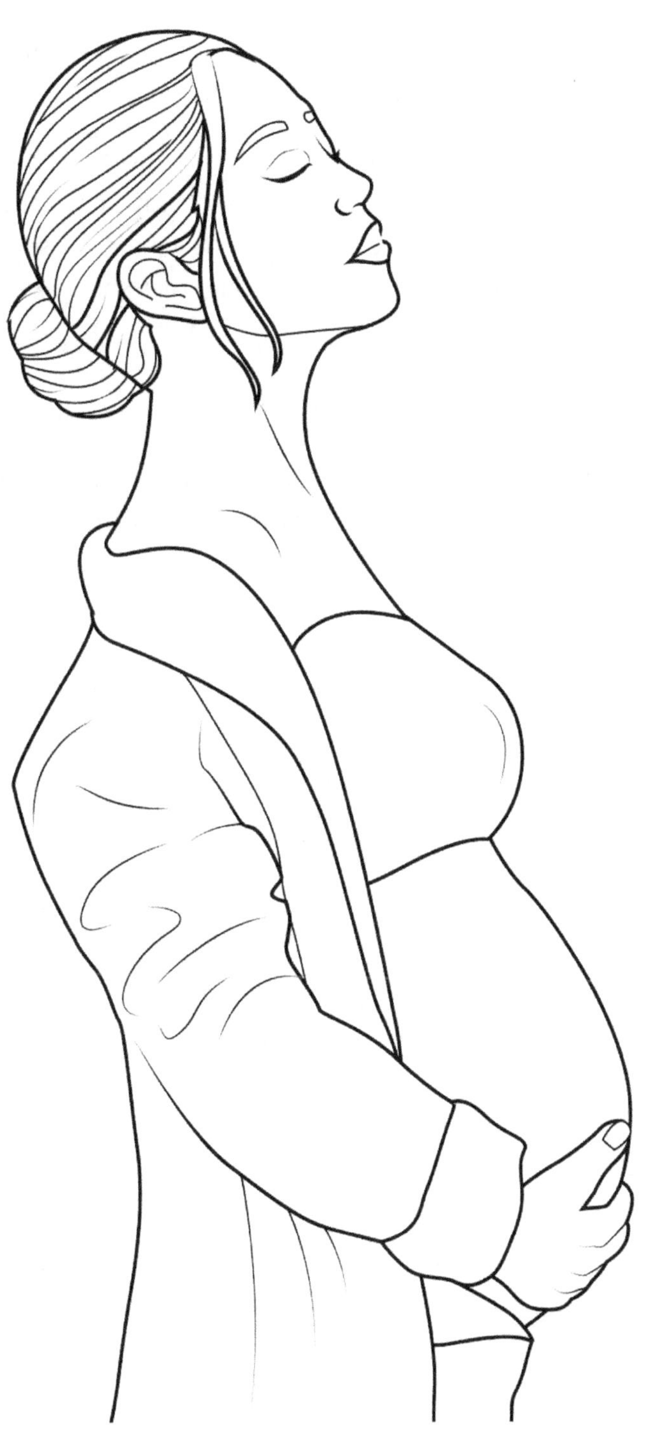

Self-health is not selfish. I'll never get tired of saying this. As busy as you are, find time to care for your changing body. In addition to sleep and nourishment, consider things like:

- Acupuncture or massage - with an experienced prenatal practitioner.

- Prenatal yoga (in-person classes can be great for meeting new moms-to-be, and online classes offer flexibility and cut down on travel-time).

- Regular physical activity (under the supervision of a knowledgeable trainer and with your physician's consent). A lot of pregnant women enjoy exercising in water for the feeling of weightlessness that provides a welcome contrast with their new normal. As with the above, make sure any instructor or trainer is aware that you are expecting. They should also be trained and experienced to help you exercise safely.

Journal prompt:

How do you relate to your body? Are those feelings carrying over from pre-pregnancy, or are they new? If these are familiar feelings, explore the potential source. If they are new, give yourself space to articulate them. Be curious.

See if you can build up a habit and incorporate it during your day – at bedtime or on your lunch break. You can even do it while driving or standing in line at the store.

Bodies at work

What adjustments do you need to make in your workplace to accommodate your changing physical needs? Some possibilities include:

- A different desk/chair setup for comfort.

- Increased breaks for movement and going to the bathroom.

- Schedule or activity changes to accommodate energy levels.

- Starting family leave before 40 weeks to allow for rest and preparation.

- A plan for experiencing contractions or going into labor at work.

Remember, the Americans with Disabilities Act protects women with a pregnancy-related disability from being terminated, demoted, or denied a promotion. For example, if you need an extension of leave due to a post-partum mood disorder, you can use this protection.

Postpartum

The baby's here—awe, joy, love, fear, excitement, and exhaustion.

These pages are here to offer you support, encouragement, and – above all – space during this whirlwind. I've kept it short and sweet, with lots of room for you to reflect, color, plan, and dream. As always (but all the more so during this intense time), take what you need and let go of the rest. Or better put: take what you need – and rest.

Emotional

What to expect with baby blues.

Normal and expected for two weeks of mood fluctuations. You might be experiencing new and changing feelings about your body, your partner, about the end of your pregnancy. You'll also be bonding with your baby – but remember, attachment takes time. Sometimes it's immediate, and sometimes it takes longer. There's no one way the mom-baby relationship should look.

Remember: When you go to your post-partum visits, you'll be asked to fill out the Edinburgh or PHQ-9 questionnaires about mood. While it might be nerve-wracking to share negative feelings with your provider, don't fear an uncomfortable conversation – or worry about getting a call from CPS if you say "yes" to any of the questions. The provider is there to monitor and support you.

Journal prompt:

Your birth story

Now is the perfect time to record your birth story while it is still fresh in your mind. It can be therapeutic to retell your story, both in written form and in conversation, with a trusted friend or your partner.

Sleep

Coloring page

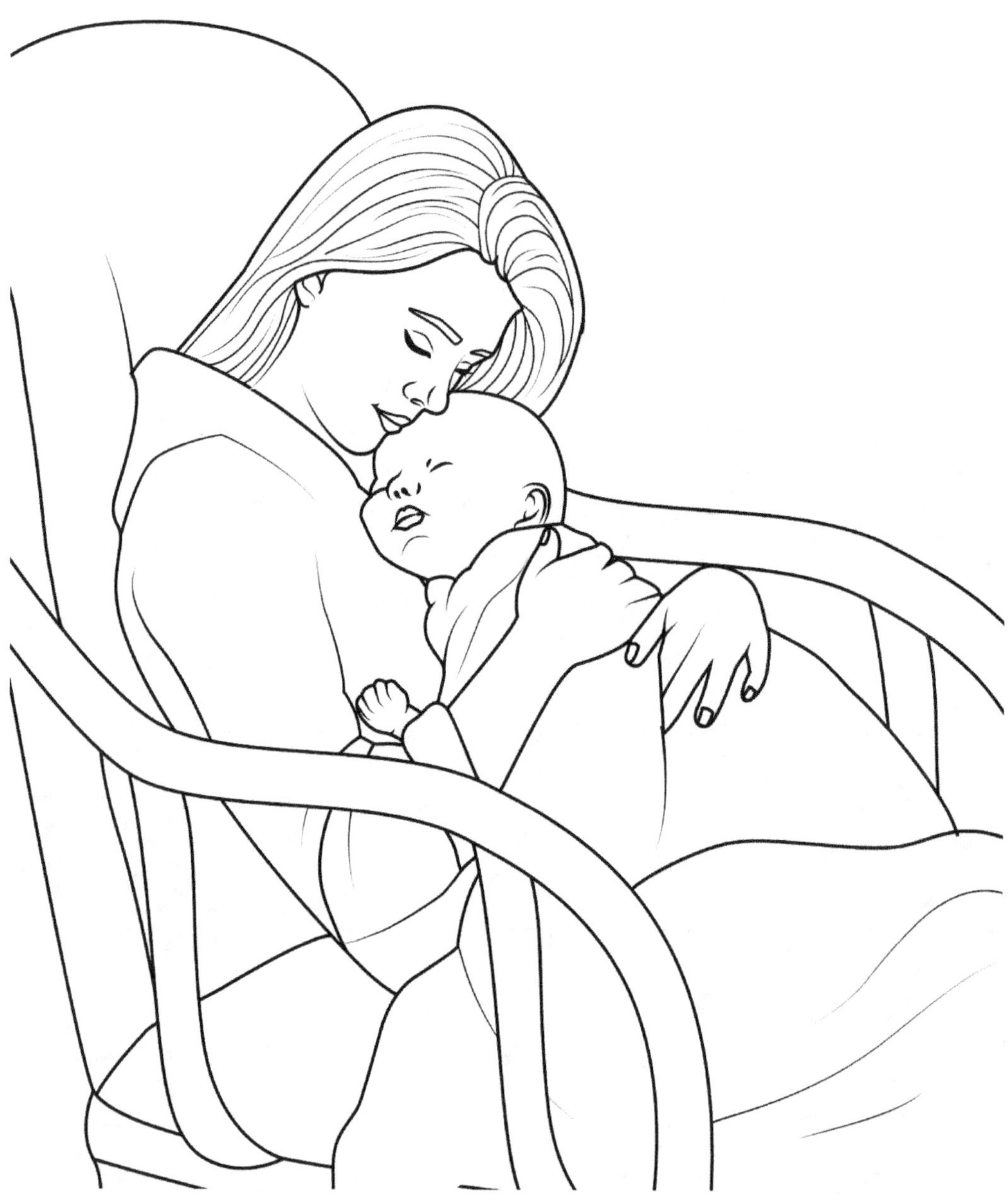

It's a brave new world when it comes to sleep. You've gone through the intense work of labor. Maybe you didn't get a wink of sleep for 72 hours or more—the adrenaline rush and cortisol spikes. You've been tired before, but now your brain is in a completely different place from the intellectual exhaustion of work. You're sleeping for shorter chunks of time between hospital wake-ups and feedings. Maybe you're coordinating NICU visits, negotiating the rhythms of your milk production, trying to discover a new comfortable position in your post-partum body. Oh, and trying to get to know your baby's sleep pattern, which could very well still be mimicking the habits of the womb.

It's objectively a lot. It's also intensely private and completely unique to your family unit. Cultural norms also play a big part in informing whether you plan to co-sleep or put your baby in their own room and bed early on. If there's a partner and/or in-laws, there will be plenty of cooks in the kitchen with their ideas of what's best for you and for the baby. Consider these pages a place for you to explore what might work best for you.

Making the bedroom a sanctuary

Shape the environment to serve you best. Consider:

- Fast access to nourishing foods and water. Your favorite water bottle and a granola bar on the nightstand can do the trick.

- Lactation supplies: a cloth to mop leaks, breast pads, and a nursing pillow.

- A sound machine, eye pillow, soothing playlist, and other comfort items.

- A dimmable bedside lamp.

- Loose, comfortable, easy-to-wash pjs.

- Easy to wash sheets.

Sleep hygiene:

- Create a bedtime routine that you can stick to as regularly as possible (light stretches, a bath, a few minutes of reading, a body scan, prayer, or meditation).

- Make your room comfortable (set a cool temperature, check on light levels, choose comfortable bedding, consider a white noise machine).

- Move throughout the day if your OB/GYN says it's okay. Walking and stretching count!

- Keep any caffeine consumption away from bedtime.

- Minimize or eliminate foods such as sugar, alcohol, and fried or spicy foods, which are known to disrupt sleep.

"Sleep when the baby sleeps." Great advice, except when it's not. Sometimes it's just not practical. Sometimes, your body won't turn off. The last thing you need is another source of guilt. Let me reframe it for you. If you can't sleep, at least rest.

Rest can look like a lot of things. Eyes closed while nursing, deep breaths when someone else picks up the baby, or a shower.

Mantras for rest

On a restless night, it can help to have many tools in your toolbox. For some people, holding onto a mantra can do the trick. Here are some suggestions of mantras for sleep, or create your own.

"Sleep will come."

"My body will take care of me."

"I can let go and rest."

____

____

____

Nutrition

As you transition between nourishing your baby inside your body and outside, remember there are still two parts to the equation: the baby and you. So much attention goes to baby's feeding: formula, breast milk, bottles, or whatever the combination might be. But you are an integral piece of the puzzle, so let's focus some attention on your top priorities during post-partum.

Whether or not you are lactating, you need to nourish yourself intentionally, to replenish from the experience of pregnancy and labor, and to fuel yourself for the effort ahead. That includes eating healthy foods and staying well hydrated.

Comfort foods are great during this time filled with emotion. At the same time, make sure to get plenty of lean proteins, complex carbohydrates, and plant-based fats (think avocado, nuts, etc.). This isn't about taking off "baby weight." It's just about giving your body a chance to heal and reset.

Support yourself and ask for support.

What are three ways you can support yourself nutritionally during this time? Number your priorities from 1-3. Use these examples or write your own.

- Drink more water

- Buy pre-cut veggies and fruit for snacking

- Keep healthy snacks on your nightstand

- Prioritize whole foods over processed

- Incorporate a regular treat in your diet

- ____

- ____

- ____

Friends and family often want to help a new parent but don't know how. What are three ways you can ask for support during this time? Number your priorities from 1-3. Use these examples or write your own.

- Request a ready-to-heat meal from __________________

- Ask __________________ to cook or do dishes for you while you nap

- Ask __________________ to pick up your take-out food order

- ____

- ____

Financial

The world may be rushing around out there, but short of immediate emergencies, leave them on the other side of the door.

Money worries

> Drop your money worries here. Get them out of your head and see if you feel a little lighter.

"Hit the snooze button"

If you've got bills coming due, put them in a pile or a folder in your inbox and out of your mind. There's almost always a 30-day grace period, so don't stress. Designate someone else to handle any of these minor financial obligations wherever possible.

"Don't mind if I do…"

Having a baby is expensive. New moms are a coveted demographic for corporations of all kinds. Don't be shy about taking advantage of all the free samples that are available as you experiment with different types of formula, diapers, creams, etc.

Childcare

At some point in the post-partum period, it's bound to happen: you separate from your baby for the first time. For some, it's in the hospital. For others, it comes later on when an eager relative offers their arms – and urges you to take some time for yourself.

Prompt:

This first "solo" experience might have been a relief; it might have raised anxiety. Maybe a little bit of both. Reflect on how you feel when others watch your baby:

____

____

____

____

____

____

Communication:

When you hand off the baby to someone else for more than just a few minutes, you're going to want to exchange information about what's been going on. I call this a 'debriefing.' It might include things about when the baby last slept and for how long, when they last ate and how much, diaper changes, any spitting up, signs of discomfort, etc. The 'debrief' will be a crucial communication piece for the working mom – especially when you return to work. Reflect on what a healthy debrief looks like to you so you can practice in these early stages.

Things I want to share about the baby when I hand them off:

1. ____

2. ____

3. ____

Things I want to know about the baby when I return:

1. ____

2. ____

3. ____

Social

The biggest hormone shift a woman experiences during the perinatal period comes in the first two post-partum weeks. Support is of the essence.

But what kind of support and when? You may have lined up visits and plans or organized a meal train during your pregnancy, and now you're looking at a very different reality than the one you imagined. As much as you look forward to being fed by other people, you dread the thought of answering the door when someone brings you a casserole at the moment that 50 other things are happening all at once, and you can't remember when you last had a shower.

That's okay. The terms of engagement are yours to set.

Prompt

- "You can best support me by…"

Your loved ones want to be helpful – and they'll likely reach out with offers that sound most helpful to them. They can only know what you need if you tell them. Practice writing out your preferred kinds of support. Maybe you want a prepared meal; maybe you'd love someone to come to your house and make you a cup of tea while you share your birth story. Maybe you'd like someone to play with your other child(ren).

Social scripts

When setting your boundaries for post-partum visits, you can consider asking your partner or trusted family member/friend to handle these comings and goings for you so that you minimize surprises and inopportune appearances.

But what about when someone arrives unannounced, or you bump into your chatty neighbor while on a quick stroll to the mailbox? It can help to develop a strategy to feel empowered to engage in the way that serves you best.

Gratitude

As much as we anticipate what our post-partum relationships will be like, there's nothing like a new baby in the house to shake everything up. Sometimes, the best interactions are small and unexpected, providing a powerful pick-me-up when stress is high.

Take a moment to express gratitude for the positive social interaction you had this week. After writing it down, consider sharing it with the person.

Physical

As you're adjusting to this new phase of your body, it's normal to experience all sorts of conflicting feelings. Awe for what you've gone through. Disappointment or anger for parts of the birth that didn't go the way you hoped. You may also experience discomfort mixed with aches and acute pains, mixed with relief. Those first few times going to the bathroom might make you feel like you're in an alien body. Learning to nurse will put you in a completely different relationship with your breasts and nipples. Your hunger and energy levels may fluctuate wildly – this is the biggest hormonal change a new mom experiences.

Gratitude

Even as we celebrate the miracle of what we've done, it's so common to feel critical of the body that enabled it all to happen. Brand new stretch marks, aches and pains, swelling, and body parts that barely resemble what we remember from before baby. A gratitude practice that includes your body may help you shift away from these negative thoughts – and allow you to develop a healthy post-partum relationship with movement.

Pick one part of your body that you are grateful for. Write it down and think about why. Be as specific as possible.

For example, I love my strong arms because they allow me to cradle my baby.

Post-partum movement tips:

Your ob/gyn will need to clear you for exercise – usually after your six-week check-up. Once that happens, get moving in whatever way feels good: stretching, foam rolling, brief walks, yoga, or a gentle return to the activity you loved before you became pregnant. Just check in with your doctor about it before getting started.

1.   Good enough is good enough. Even five minutes of gentle movement can be enough for where your body is right now, so be kind to yourself if that's what exercise looks like right now. If you had an active lifestyle pre-baby, it might feel strange, but it won't always be this way. This is a time to get to know yourself in a new way, so save yourself some sweat and take it easy.

2.   Prioritize healing. Physical therapy, pelvic floor therapy, and even massage therapy. These are all ways to reconnect to your body in the post-partum period.

3.   Use the childcare at your gym. Many gyms offer free childcare, usually for babies older than six weeks. This can be a win-win – a way to practice separating from your baby while staying nearby and caring for yourself. (Pro-tip: Your partner can also take the baby to the gym with them, leaving you some well-deserved "me time.")

4.   Make it a team sport. You might feel hesitant to call on your support people for more help to do something like exercise. But exercise is a crucial part of well-being, not a luxury. Those endorphins will help fill your cup, which will, in turn, help you care for everyone who depends on you.

Pre Transition Back to Work

Emotional

Depending on how long your maternity leave is, you may find yourself in this "pre-transitional" moment while your c-section scars are still fresh – or after you've spent weeks and months developing a new routine with your little one.

Regardless of when your transition is taking place, it is not uncommon for new moms to start feeling an increased sense of urgency in the final days and weeks. There is so much to do objectively – on a practical level but also an emotional level. You may feel a sense of mourning as you say goodbye to certain routines and habits. You may also feel a sense of excitement and relief. You may feel pulled in eighty directions at once.

The important thing is that you make room for those emotions. While you go about your day – and fill every hour to the brim – you want to strike a balance. Yes, putting in a little extra preparation now may set you up for success in this new life phase, but you don't want to dive into emotional avoidance by working around the clock. Allow yourself to enjoy the end of your leave without feeling the urge to overcompensate for your time off or make up for reduced 'productivity.'

Yellow flags:

A stagnant emotional state, feeling robotic, numb, mechanical, or like you're just going through the motions.

Tip: Set a reminder for yourself every hour to do a 60-second body scan or try box breathing. Even something as simple as focusing on your feet and making contact with the ground can help calm the limbic system.

Sleep

Take a deep breath. Sleep will be top of mind for you during this period – your shut-eye will become even more precious as you prepare for your return to work, and you'll also be thinking about how your baby's sleep will change: they might have to adjust to a group nap schedule at a daycare center; they might have to go down for a nap with a different caregiver, like a nanny or another family member.

You might be asking questions about sleep training and how it fits with the return to work – is now the time to do it? You and your partner might have different experiences and ideas around sleep, making these decisions more complicated.

Take another deep breath. You may feel tempted to hire a fancy sleep consultant or buy every book and product on the market promising to make your baby sleep like an angel. I recommend you take a hot minute, take (yet) another deep breath, reach out to your network for help, and, if possible, take a nap.

Planning for sleep transition

If you already have a return-to-work date on the calendar, you may want to do a little advance planning around sleep transitions. Often, sleep training occurs around six months, which coincidentally can be a time when your baby starts teething – and when you are headed back to work.

There's no one-size-fits-all, so the best advice I can give is to plan ahead – and to plan in some flexibility around that plan. If you plan to sleep train, but those teeth start poking up, give yourself permission to adapt.

Depending on your work situation, you may want to create a 'crisis plan' to address what happens if sleep goes off the rails and you need shut-eye to function the next day. That might mean discussing in advance with a partner, securing the help of a relative, or looking into a night nanny to take some shifts.

Above all, your pediatrician is the expert on sleep, so don't be afraid to ask questions (and then ask more questions).

Interrupted sleep is objectively problematic. But sometimes, internal stressors might be making things feel worse. The next exercise will help get those stressors out into the open.

Sleep beliefs

Sleep can feel so natural that we forget to look at the experiences and beliefs that condition our ideas about sleep (or lack of sleep). Take some time to reflect on yours, and if you have a partner, ask them to do the same. Share your answers with each other, giving each person uninterrupted time to speak.

____

____

____

____

____

Nutrition

One of the best ways you can help yourself in anticipation of your transition back is to spend time thinking about your nutrition game plan.

When I say game plan, I do not mean you need to become a Michelin-star chef or a kitchen influencer. What I do mean is to figure out how to streamline your time in the kitchen and grocery store so that it works for you and your family. If you don't have a game plan, you may end up with take-out every night, which won't be sustainable long-term.

Things to think about – family meals.

- What kind of division of labor can you devise with your partner, if you have one?

For example, assign each person different days of the week for cooking or divide mealtime chores (planning, shopping, prepping, cooking, and cleaning).

- What kinds of tools/products can you incorporate into your cooking to simplify? (crockpot, pre-chopped or frozen produce, etc.)

- What kinds of easy, fast meals do you want to try? (One-pot dishes, sheet pan meals, no-cook charcuterie boards, giant salad with protein)

- Are there healthy meal delivery, hot food bar options (usually better than take-out!), or healthy/convenient take-out options?

- How can I incorporate meal prep sessions (1-2x per week) to save time in the kitchen? (Think: large batches of soups and stews, crockpot meals)

- Whom can I incorporate in my nutrition game plan (relatives, friends, neighbors, other household members)?

Write down your three best ideas.

1. ____

2. ____

3. ____

Things to think about – daytime meals

Eating at work will look different for every mama. So much depends on your workplace setup, responsibilities, and schedule. You may need to get creative, so ask around – other mamas and other people in your workplace or career might have ideas on how to incorporate healthy eating into the workday.

Breastfeeding/pumping mamas may want to have a one-time consultation with a post-partum nutritionist who can recommend how to eat to support and protect your milk supply.

- What kinds of dishes can I make that work as lunchtime leftovers?

- What are the healthy, convenient options available at/near work?

- Do I have a good quality lunch bag and water bottle for the office?

- What healthy snacks should I bring with me?

(Bars and packaged foods can be great options; just look for products with whole food ingredients, and watch out for high levels of sodium and added sugar)

- Think beyond 'snacks.' Oatmeal cups, healthy soups, a small portion of a regular meal can all be 'snacks.'

Write down your three best ideas.

1. ____

2. ____

3. ____

Things to think about – baby

- If the baby is starting to eat table food during this time, how do you plan to introduce solids? (Find a trusted brand, prep/freeze simple homemade purees, etc.)

- If your baby will be taking a bottle with a caregiver, now's the time to ensure they get used to bottles. Many babies will be particular about the nipple they prefer, so plan to buy lots of different brands until you find the one you like (and don't buy a lot of the same one until you know they'll take it).

Reframe

Food is close to the heart. There's also so much societal baggage that goes along with feeding your family and being a working mom. On top of the pressure to feed your family, there's also the "get your 'old' body back" narrative that often screams loudly during this time. I'd like to invite you to construct thoughts and affirmations around feeding your body for nourishment and sustainability, whatever that looks like to you.

If negative thoughts arise around nourishing yourself, try a reframe to see them in a positive light.

I need to get my diet back in shape so I can lose the baby weight →. Healthy eating habits will allow me to fuel myself during this busy season.

Financial

To budget or not to budget?

That is a question I will not attempt to answer. I'll ask: Is your current financial situation working for you (and your partner if you have one)?

Audit

During this transitional time, your needs might change dramatically; your values, on the other hand, might stay rock solid – or there might be perspective shifts there as well. You'll certainly have new and different expenses to consider – and perhaps changes in your income.

If you have a budget, this is a great opportunity to reassess. Ask yourself:

- How can your budget better meet your needs?

____

____

____

- What are the new or returning budget items (commuting costs, daycare, diapers, etc.)?

____

____

____

- Where are the places you can save? (hooray for tax credits)

____

____

____

- Where are the areas where you want to invest? (college savings, vacation fund, home down payment, rainy day fund)

____

____

____

If you don't have a budget but want to try, I recommend looking at popular apps that break down spending into categories and give you charts and graphs around trends.

Childcare

It's time to get your ducks in a row.

That includes creating a back-up or emergency plan. Daycares close, kiddos get sick, nannies have emergencies, work runs late, and traffic gets out of control – sometimes at the absolute least convenient time. Expect the unexpected.

Depending on your work obligations (and your partner's, if you have one), the back-up plan might need to change week by week, but if you stay on top of your options, you're more likely to know what to do in a pinch.

Things to consider:

- What are the daycare/nanny's policies around illness?

- How do you handle late pick-ups?

- What are unmovable appointments for each of you?

- When can each parent be 'on-call'?

- Who can provide back-up care (family, neighbors, other parents)?

- What is your office policy on sick days? Does your employer offer back-up childcare for emergencies? Are children allowed in the workplace in emergencies?

- How will work expect you to handle emergency situations?

Social

As you prepare to return to work, you're getting ready for some level of social transition. You may feel separation anxiety about spending less time with your baby. You may have to bow out of groups that have become part of your weekly social fabric, like mommy & me classes, storytime, or mom-baby yoga.

You will also form new relationships or return to old ones – your childcare provider will be a major figure in your life, as will your professional contacts. Use this transitional moment to think about these relationships and what you envision for them in the future.

Audit: Cup-fillers and cup-drainers

With limited energy and so much on your plate, the last thing you need is extra drama.

Which relationships fill your cup? How can you nourish them?

Which relationships drain you? How can you set appropriate boundaries?

Connecting with important figures

The best way to ensure strong relationships is to communicate intentionally. Use this space to think about how you want to approach communication with major figures.

- Your child: What kind of rituals can you incorporate into your day as you say goodbye and reunite? What objects can help ease the transition for both of you? (A photo album for you to scroll through; a blanket with your smell for them to nap with)

- Childcare provider: What will your pre/post-care debrief look like? Is communication in person or via an app? What information needs to be exchanged?

- Partner communication: What's the best way to get a hold of your partner during the workday? In emergencies? Can you set up a recurring 'meeting' time to address longer topics? Can you incorporate a daily or nightly ritual? (Something simple. Sharing a bedtime snack counts!)

- Colleagues/supervisors: Be mindful of how people are treating you on the way back. If you don't establish clear boundaries and expectations, they'll only have assumptions to fall back on. Do you want communication before your first day back, and if so, how? What level of involvement do you want?

Physical

During this transitional time, a return to movement will be a big help. Exercise gets endorphins flowing, and depending on where you choose to move, you can use physical activity as a chance to be in nature, spend time with your baby, hang out with (or make new) friends, or have alone time.

Journal prompt:

How do you want to relate to your body during this transitional time? In what ways can you care for your body as you prepare for your return to work?

Remember, movement doesn't mean training for the next Olympics (unless that's your thing). It could mean having a three-minute PJ dance party, a stroll to the grocery store, an online yoga video, or anything else that gets your heart pumping. Post-pandemic, there are infinite options for online/home workouts, in addition to more traditional gyms, martial arts classes, etc.

As you ease back into movement, I recommend:

- Looking for programs/trainers with specific post-partum knowledge and training, especially if you are starting something new.

- Exercise to feel good and honor your body, not to force it back into shape.

- Choose something you love.

- Ease in gradually.

- Incorporate stretching and recovery exercises (foam rolling) no matter what kind of exercise you choose.

- Bring your baby if you want. There are groups such as "stroller strides" that incorporate babies into workouts. Mom-baby post-natal yoga classes or videos can also be a fun way to get back into movement together.

Audit:

Clothes & accessories for back-to-work

Check your closet: What do you need to get back to work? Don't try to squeeze into your pre-baby clothes. Buy a few comfy staples in your current size (thrift shops are great for this kind of shopping, as are 'buy-nothing' groups). Flexible waistbands are your friend.

If you're pumping in the office, look for a few dark-colored nursing tops or patterns (in case of leakage/stains). You'll also want comfy breast pads (disposable or washable) and nursing bras if you don't have them yet.

Reframe

The thought of returning to work may have brought up feelings about how your body is now versus pre-baby. Write down any negative thoughts and then consider a positive reframe:

My old body is 'gone.' → My body has gained wisdom from this experience.

Early Back to Work

Emotional

There aren't enough words to describe the emotional complexity of the back-to-work period, not to mention the diversity of experiences. You may be elated, exhausted, anxious, invigorated, numb, or all – or none – of the above.

For some of you, this back-to-work period is happening when your baby is in their first few days, weeks or months of life. You might have developed a longstanding routine – and still feel like it wasn't long enough. You might feel rushed out the door or impatient to return to work.

For those mamas who are experiencing separation anxiety, I want to say I see you. For some of you, anxiety might be a familiar state of mind. For others, it might feel like a new, unwelcome visitor. Speak to a trusted medical professional if you are experiencing anxiety (separation or otherwise).

Here are some ways to help ease the transition.

Try transitional objects: sleep with a shirt or blanket you can leave with your nanny or daycare provider so your baby smells your scent throughout the day or during naptime.

Create rituals for drop off and pick up: you might sing a certain song, plan to breastfeed immediately upon arrival at daycare or have a special greeting.

Make yourself mementos: Have pictures or a phone photo album easily accessible to look at throughout the day, especially while you are pumping.

Use live updates wisely: Some daycares or nannies will provide live updates. If you have this possibility, be mindful about how you want to use it. (Staring at a webcam from 9-5 never helped anyone.) Maybe a 5-minute check-in twice a day? What would help you?

"My best is enough."

As you enter this new phase, take time to decide on gentle, compassionate affirmations to lean on when things get tough. A traffic jam, an unexpected daycare closing, a surprise assignment at work, or your baby's first sickness. These are all common for the course.

You may also be tempted to make comparisons with others around you. It's only natural. We're a social species. "Everyone makes it look so easy." "They must have something I don't." Nine times out of ten, those people are plagued by the same doubts.

Let go of these self-judgements and focus on self-compassion.

Examples of affirmations:

"This is hard, but I can do hard things."

"My best is enough."

...

Thoughts-feelings-behavior

The cognitive behavioral triangle recognizes – and works to shift – the interplay between thoughts, feelings, and behavior. Here's an example: Cindy, your coworker, is reaching out to you a week before your return date, asking you a work-related question.

- Thought: "How rude. Cindy knows I'm not back for another week."

- Feelings: Anger, frustration.

- Behavior: A curt response.

If you shift any one of those things, you can change the others. For example, a thought like, "Cindy values my input on the team," can lead to feelings of appreciation and more positive (or neutral) behavior.

Create your own triangle here to work through a difficult situation:

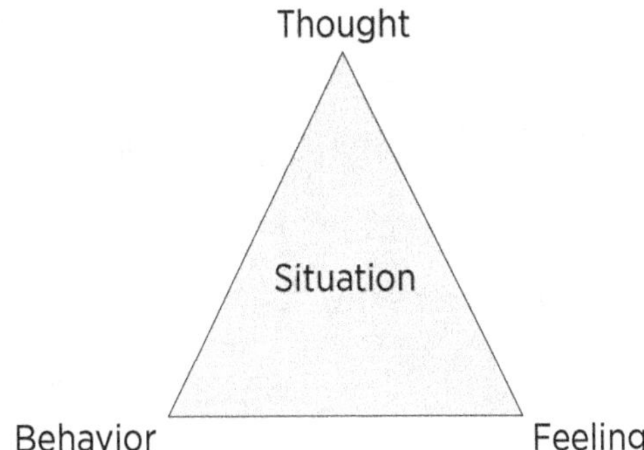

<u>Setting priorities / letting go of perfection</u>

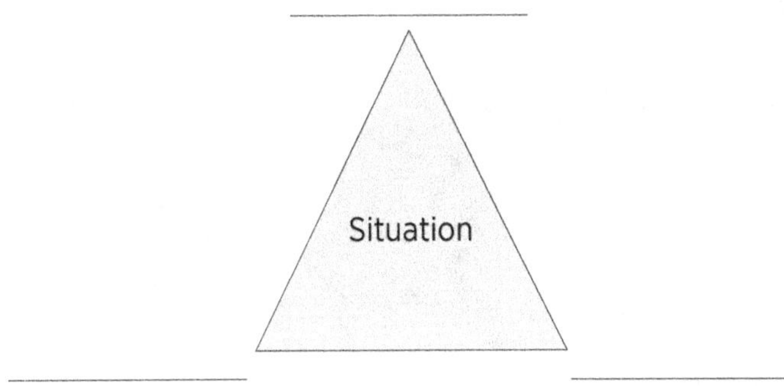

Sleep

Self-compassion will come in handy in the sleep department as you transition to childcare. Naps may be a challenge. They may need to shift depending on the provider's schedule and the baby's development. You may also have changing needs to accommodate your new schedule and energy requirements. Consider sleep a work in progress, and prioritize planning for sleep shifts with your partner if you have one and your childcare provider.

"Partner renegotiation"

I invite both you and your partner to take time to consider the following questions individually.

- When you're at your best, what does sleep look like?

____

____

____

- What is the minimum you need to function?

____

____

____

- Now, sit down and look over your respective answers. Give each partner time to share without interruption. Then reflect:

____

____

____

What changes can you make? Consider any of the following, and brainstorm additional solutions of your own:

- Changes to bedtime or routine.

- Changes to bedtime duties (who wakes up for feedings, what nights).

- Hiring an occasional night nanny or asking for support from a relative.

- Considerations on where the baby is sleeping now versus where you would like them to sleep.

What are your 2-3 best solutions?

1. ____

____

____

2. ____

____

____

3. ____

____

What immediate steps will you take to put them into practice? (Be as concrete as possible.)

What, if anything, do you need to resolve in order to move ahead?

"Sleepy affirmations"

After months of being woken up by your baby, the unthinkable might happen: a middle-of-the-night wake-up all on your own as your baby sleeps soundly. I hear a lot of worry, disappointment, and frustration around this scenario as if it is a sign the sleep routine has been permanently altered. I know that a lost night of sleep can feel like a gut punch. But I like to invite mamas to put these nights into perspective.

What thoughts go through your brain when you wake up without your baby?

How can you reframe them? For example, "My body will relearn a more steady sleep schedule" or "I can use this time to pump and build up my milk supply."

If you have other thoughts about sleep that are no longer serving you, write them below.

Brain dump

Now, think about how you can reframe them to meet your needs better. (Consider posting your affirmations near your bed for easy night-time access.)

Negative thoughts on sleep	Positive reframe
My baby is a 'bad' sleeper.	This, too, shall pass.
Nights are stressful.	I can face what the night brings.
My baby will never let me sleep.	Rest will come.

Now, rewrite your narrative from this new perspective.

Positive revision

____

____

____

____

____

____

____

Strategies for the sleepless night

If I had one piece of advice for parents on a sleepless night, it's this:

This is not the rest of your life. It's just one night.

When you are sleep-deprived, irrational thinking tends to take over. During the night, see where you can introduce some perspective with a self-soothing internal dialog: take one moment at a time.

Tips for the next day

Be strategic with what work you do (do mindless tasks when sleep-deprived - if possible).

Power nap when possible.

Stay hydrated.

Be gentle with yourself as you head into bedtime.

Use your support and tools for the next night: If you have a partner or family member, ask them to cover the next night. If you've talked to your doctor about a sleep aid, it might be the time to put it to use.

Nutrition

Back to work means a new relationship to food, for better and for worse. Maybe your meal train is over, and now you need to organize your meals yourself. But maybe you actually have time for a meal for the first time since your baby's arrival. Now's a great time to take a beat and think about how you're doing and how you want to shape your nutrition going forward.

Audit

Celebrate the wins. Check your perfectionism at the door. Be gentle with yourself and recognize you're doing the best you can. List the things that are going well that you want to continue and expand.

What could be going better, food-wise? What one thing can you add, eliminate, or change going into this week to improve your nutrition?

____

____

____

____

____

____

____

____

____

What's your food-mood relationship?

Food can be a tool and a resource, but when we're running on fumes, it seems easier to reach for the extra candy bar, drink another coffee, and just keep going.

Use this space to reflect on how your diet impacts your mood. Experiment: If you eat more brain-powered food like Omegas or incorporate lean protein into your diet, do you see an impact on your productivity and energy?

Things I've noticed about my food-mood relationship.

____

____

____

____

____

____

____

____

____

____

____

____

____

What are the top 5 foods that make you feel better – not just while they're in your mouth, but in the hours after you eat them?

1. ____

2. ____

3. ____

4. ____

5. ____

Which foods do you want to moderate?

1. ____

2. ____

3. ____

4. ____

5. ____

Which foods do you want to avoid? (Think trigger foods that are hard to eat in small portions, especially highly processed foods).

1. ____

2. ____

3. ____

4. ____

5. ____

Financial

Okay, you've sent in that first daycare payment or handed your nanny a large check; I get it. That drain on your paycheck is hard. I've had plenty of conversations with moms who start rethinking whether it's worth it to stay at work when child care takes such a huge bite out of their take-home pay.

But remember, you're playing a long-term game. Your child will not be in daycare forever. This is an investment in your professional development. Take a deep breath and recognize this season is temporary.

On the one hand, moms can feel guilty about spending money on child care. On the other hand, many spend money to assuage the guilt they feel because they're sending their child to day care.

In today's media environment, advertisers capitalize on that guilt and make us think we need to buy things to fix it. The latest and greatest stroller. The most expensive thermometer in the store. Seven of your child's favorite lovey to always have on hand.

Here's a gentle reminder: be mindful of impulse purchases, whether it comes from fear around a first cold or jealousy that other parents have the latest-and-greatest gadget that makes their child's life perfect.

When you feel an urge to buy something, pause. Write down the thing you want and why. Wait a few days (or at least a few hours). Then, come back and check and see if the urge has passed.

What I want	Why I want it

Childcare

For most families, the start of a new childcare situation is full of curveballs. But as things settle down, it can be helpful to have a routine in mind that takes into consideration everyone's needs. That said, I invite you to let this routine guide you, not one more thing you have to live up to. Routines get thrown off (and restored), and they also evolve. Use this space to brainstorm and dream about how a day might look.

Parts of the routine might include:

- Drop off/pick up rituals, with songs, phrases, or gestures to say goodbye to your baby and welcome each other back.

- A reunion feeding.

- Routines for the drive, including music or a phone call to a relative.

- A 30-second visualization exercise for you to center yourself prior to pick-up.

- A plan for communication with the provider (debrief on feedings and naps).

- Back-up supplies in the car: snacks (for you!), change of clothes, extra diapers.

For people who work from home and/or have childcare at home, remember that routines are still helpful in delineating the boundaries between work and home. You may not have a daily commute, but consider opportunities for incorporating intentional transitions with the start of your work day and your child's 'school' day.

Design your routine

What might a healthy routine look like for you? Who needs to be involved on each day of the week?

____

____

____

____

____

____

____

____

____

____

____

____

Social

It's a whole new world, socially. You've got new environments for social connection but also so many more stressors that might strain existing relationships.

A new working mom knows this is true: Time is truly finite. There's no time for toxic people or unpleasant spaces. Ask yourself: Who are the people you want to lean into? No time for toxic people or spaces.

Prompt: Nurturing old relationships

Think of a relationship you value highly (partner, relative, friend, colleague) and consider how you can nurture it during this major life transition.

What does 'socializing' look like now?

Time to be creative and flexible. Before your baby, you might have been able to enjoy a 4-hour paella dinner on the beach at 8 pm. Now, you might need to squeeze in a 30-minute coffee before work or a walk-and-talk. Think through your important social dynamics and how you might recreate them in your current situation, with a focus on holding onto the part of the relationship you truly value (great conversation, trust, outdoor time, etc.). Be creative.

Opening new doors

What are the new environments for social connection?	Who are the people you want to connect with?

Physical

For anyone feeling guilty about not working out enough during this period, let me validate you: there are not enough hours in the day to do everything.

Exercise snacks may be your best friend at this stage – tiny bursts of exercise (think 2-3 minutes) spread throughout the day. Studies even suggest that these regular snacks are more effective for overall wellness than an extended workout.

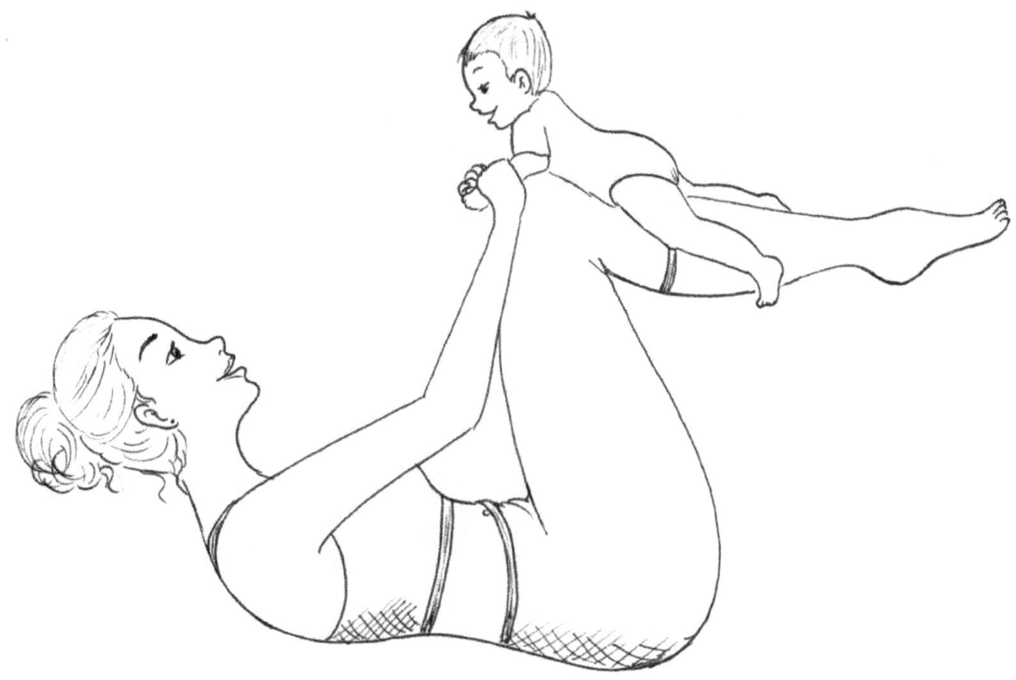

What is fun for you? What is convenient? Let go of expectations and preconceived notions of what a workout should look like.

You could:

- Have a private dance party between meetings.

- Take the stairs instead of the elevator.

- Do some desk stretches like shoulder rolls.

- Follow short online videos with simple exercise routines.

- Get a friend, colleague, or family member involved.

Add any other fun ideas for getting your body moving in a healthy way.

Settling In

Emotional

"What is your why?"

The to-do lists are long, and the days are short. From a get-it-done perspective, being a working mom can feel like a hamster wheel. It's not uncommon to hear new working moms ask, "Why am I doing all this just to pay someone else to take care of my kid?"

Now that you're in the 'settling in' phase, I invite you to reflect on the positives of working motherhood – for you and for your baby. Remember, your baby is benefitting from increased attachment figures, new friends, and new experiences, which will likely ease their future transitions to pre-k and full-time school. They are also growing up with you as a model – an example of a person who contributes to her family and her workplace.

You may also be developing new relationships with other working moms – and in the coming years, you'll be able to pay it forward to the next mom in the office or your professional group.

I also want to take this time to tell you that it won't always feel this hard. After the first year or so, most moms find themselves able to catch their breath more regularly. It can be hard to see the forest for the trees, but believe me when I say it won't be this hard forever. To help shift into this perspective, the following exercises will guide you through prompts to reflect on the long-term benefits of working motherhood, how to celebrate wins (big and small), and how to cultivate a sense of gratitude for all the beautiful mess that is working motherhood.

Journal prompt

What does it mean to you to be a working mom? What benefits have you found personally and professionally? What benefits do you think your baby is experiencing?

____

____

____

____

____

Sleep

I'm sure I'm not breaking any news here: Sleep regressions happen, sometimes for a reason like teething, other times for no reason we can see. (Again, your pediatrician can be a great resource.) In addition to the baby's challenges, you might be having trouble of your own. It can be frustrating when the baby sleeps through the night, and you're counting sheep.

Sleep is so individual, but it's also non-negotiable. Wherever you're at, take time to pause and consider.

Audit:

What's going well, and what could improve? Think about things you can control and/or tweak. Questions to consider:

- Where is the baby sleeping?

- Where do you want them to sleep?

- If they are nursing, are they night nursing? Is that okay with you? Do they need the night feed nutritionally? How can you change either the feeding schedule or the feeding method (bottle with pumped milk or formula) to help your sleep?

Nutrition

Food can be a source of joy and (often at the same time) a source of stress. Dinnertime, in particular, can be a challenge for working families. That 5:00-6:30 window when the traditional workday ends can feel like a pressure cooker: meal prep, eating, quality time, and bedtime routines all squished into precious few minutes.

Take the pressure off. This is the time for a "good enough" approach to nutrition. Plan to tweak the system later, if needed, but now is not the time to strive for chef-of-the-year. Be gentle with yourself.

Remember: the situation is fluid, and it's supposed to be evolving. If it feels chaotic and out of control, that's because it's part of the season. The baby is just learning about food. Maybe they're picky. There are so many milestones between teething and solids and more. How could it not be chaotic?

If there's a perfectionist living within you, see if you can use this time to collect data: What works and what doesn't? Do you need separate meal times for parents and baby? Do you need a take-out night? Are there ways to simplify your routine? Start with an audit and go from there.

Audit:

(Consider these questions individually and then as a couple if you have a partner.)

How is food shopping, meal prep, and clean up going? What is your current division of labor? What, if anything, needs to be changed?

How is mealtime in your family? What areas are working well? Beyond the food, can you incorporate grounding rituals into your mealtime – like sharing daily gratitude or celebration for a quick, easy pick-me-up?

Action:

*What is the number one thing about mealtime that you want to celebrate or expand?

*What is the number one thing you want to change in your nutrition going forward?

*What one step can you take to move in this direction?

Financial

Welcome to your new normal. Childcare payments are no longer new-news, and with any luck, you've taken care of the major purchases. On the other hand, your budget might have reconfigured naturally: you may not be taking a major vacation or eating out quite as often, which can balance against an increase in groceries and diaper bills.

Now is a great time to check in with your bank account (and your partner) to see if your budget is in line with your spending and your values.

Where do you want to allocate more money, for example, entertainment, help around the house, a new work wardrobe that actually fits, professional help (like a trainer, nutritionist, or therapist), or self-care?

____

____

____

Where can you cut back?

____

____

____

Identify areas of agreement and start from there.

We plan to:

____

____

____

____

____

Childcare

When you're first getting started, childcare can feel like anything but a choice. But as you settle into your situation, it's possible you'll find it offers long-term benefits beyond the immediate need. Your childcare providers may well become attachment figures in your child's life, allowing them to build meaningful connections with people beyond the immediate household. They can also support your parenting journey: the proverbial village that present-day society can sorely lack.

Audit: Is your childcare balanced?

Who is part of your childcare team? What friends, family, or community members play a part? What do they offer? (emergency pick-ups, date nights, occasional playdates, babysitting exchanges, etc.)

Do you lean more heavily on one kind of support (family versus friends, etc.)? If so, why? Is there a way to diversify the members of your childcare team?

Social

Congratulations, you've come up for air. It's a great time to look around at your social circle and think about how things are evolving – with your new parent friends, caregivers, long-term friends, and even your partner. You might consider rekindling or revitalizing relationships that have had to take a backseat during the perinatal period.

Remember, in this phase of life, you're laying the groundwork for relationships that will project into the future. That playdate you arrange today might be with your child's lifelong best friend. That babysitter you hire today might become a long-time family confidant.

Audit:

Make a list of the most significant people in your life and think about the state of your relationship. Where would you like to invest more effort? What might that look like? (A weekly walk with a friend, a date night with a partner, or a monthly phone call with a loved one far away). After you brainstorm on your own, bring them into the conversation.

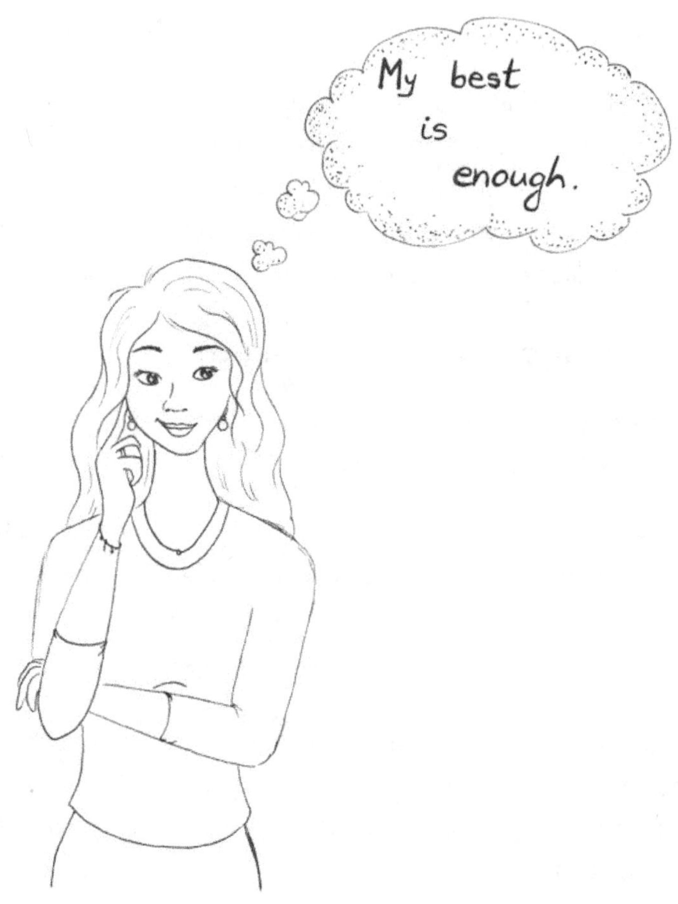

Physical

First things first: Pregnancy and lactation can wreak havoc on your body, but we often dismiss any "off" feelings because we are (of course!) exhausted. If you continue to feel low-energy or different from your usual self, check with a physician. Consider getting blood work to rule out any deficiencies or imbalances. A daily multivitamin can do wonders.

Above all, use this time to think about building habits – not just to get you through the transition (although that's good, too!), but habits for the long game.

One of the best ways to build lasting habits is to be intrinsically motivated by something deeply personal. It's different to say, "I want to go to the gym because I want to fit into my favorite jeans," versus, "I want to be healthy so that I can play with my kids without being tired."

This last exercise will help you think about the' why' for you.

"My body, my why."

Journal prompt

As a working mom, you ask your body to do so much. Your baby and your family ask your body to do so much. On top of that, society has its opinions about what women's bodies should do and how they should look.

It's not always possible to turn off those requests, those urgent demands. But let's take some space at the end of this book to focus on: What are your priorities for your body? What is your 'why' as you approach your physical health?

How can you translate that 'why' into habits? What things might you be inspired to do if you were able to focus on your 'why'?

Final thoughts

Congratulations, Mama. You've gone through some big experiences and taken time to reflect on your challenges and joys. That is worth celebrating. I feel privileged and honored that you allowed me to guide you through the ups and downs.

We've gone through the main phases of the perinatal period, but I'm the first to say that there are infinitely more things to cover. I've tried to hit the highlights here, both in terms of the big-picture issues I hear about in my practice and in terms of the concrete details, approaches, and strategies I recommend to others (and use myself). For those of you who want more in-depth reading, I've also created a full-length book on the subject, *Employed Motherhood*.

I hope the end of this workbook leads to a new chapter in our conversation about working mothers. Any of these activities can be done multiple times, so I've included some blanks in an appendix for you to return to (with more downloadable PDFs available on my website). Take what resonates with you. Please share it with your partner, family, friends, or fellow employed mamas.

Please reach out if I can be of any help to you. I'd love to hear about your experience with employed motherhood or this book. You can find me at beckygleedlmft.com.

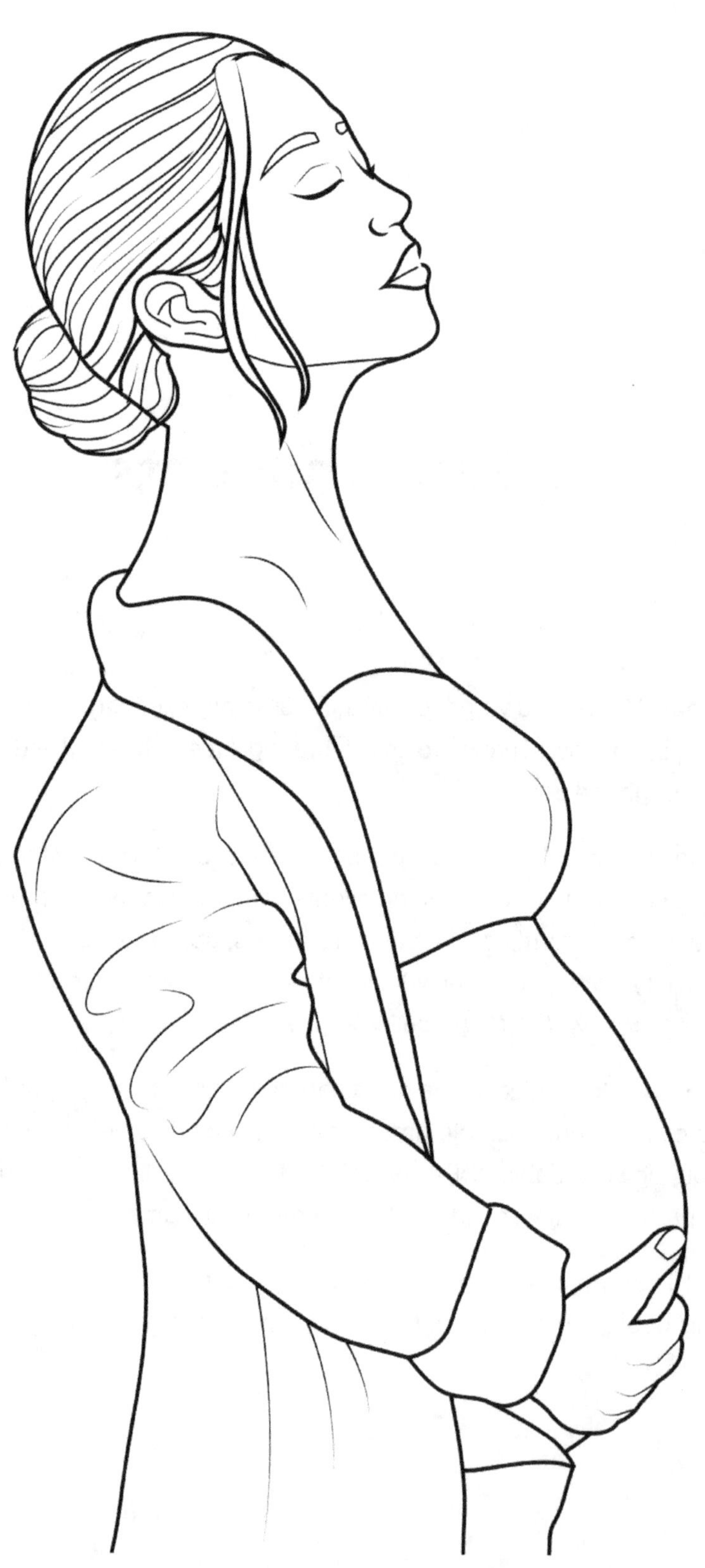

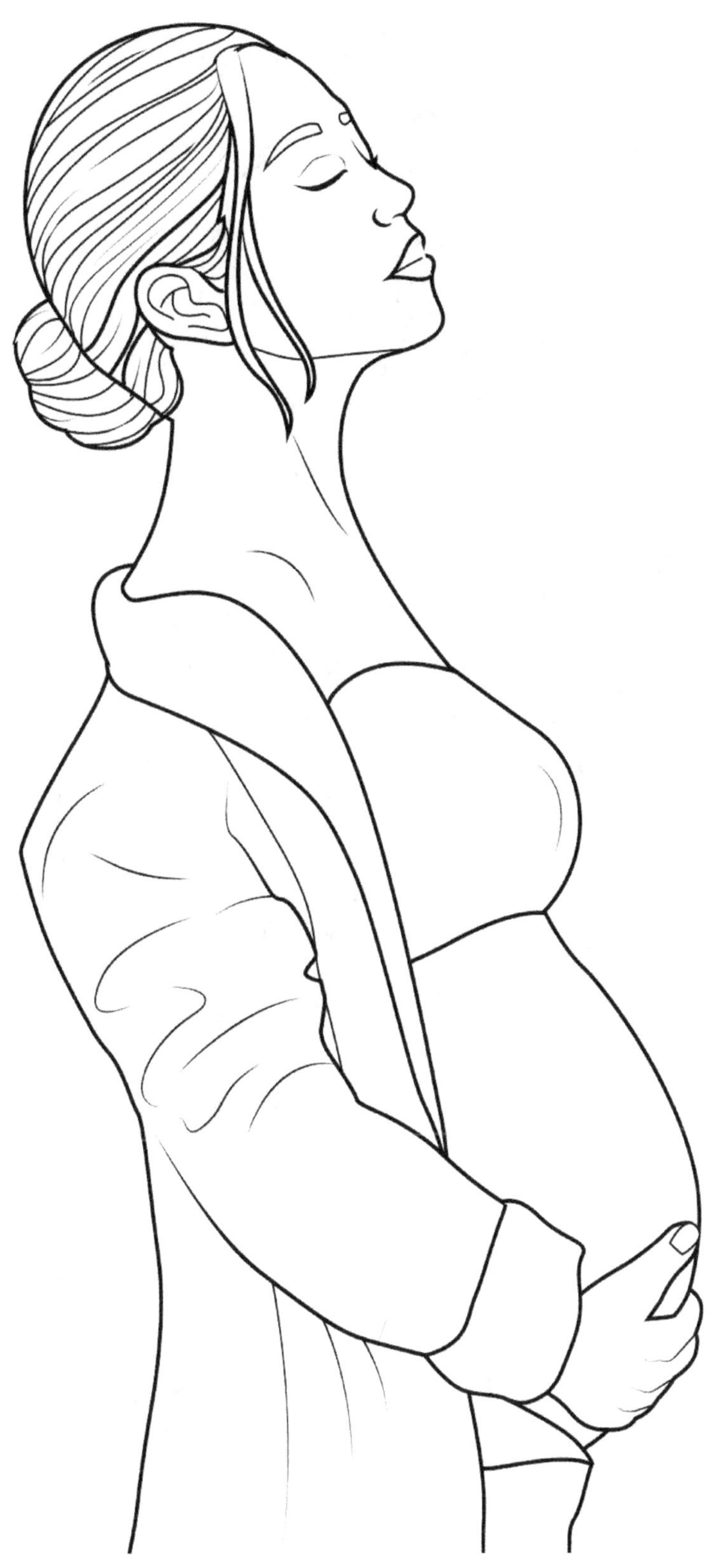

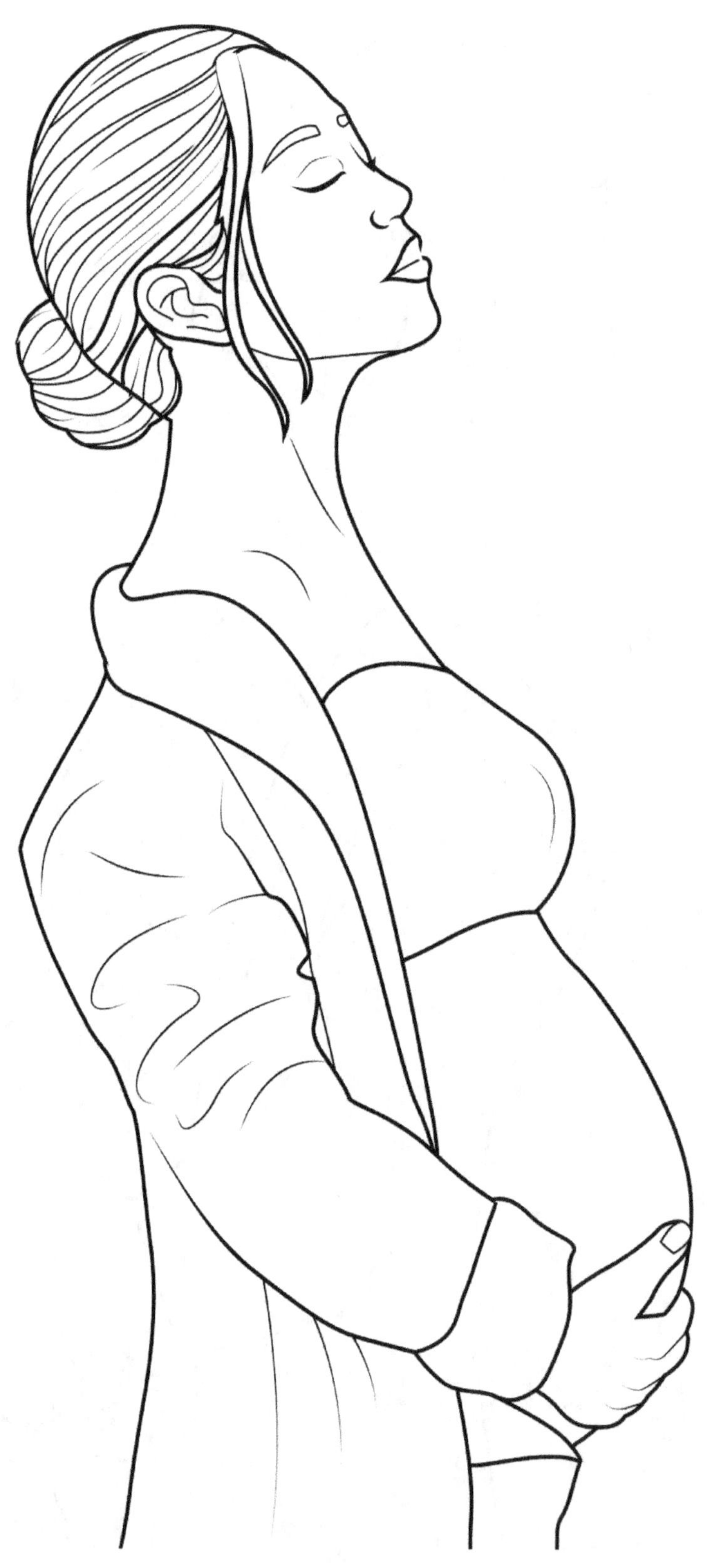

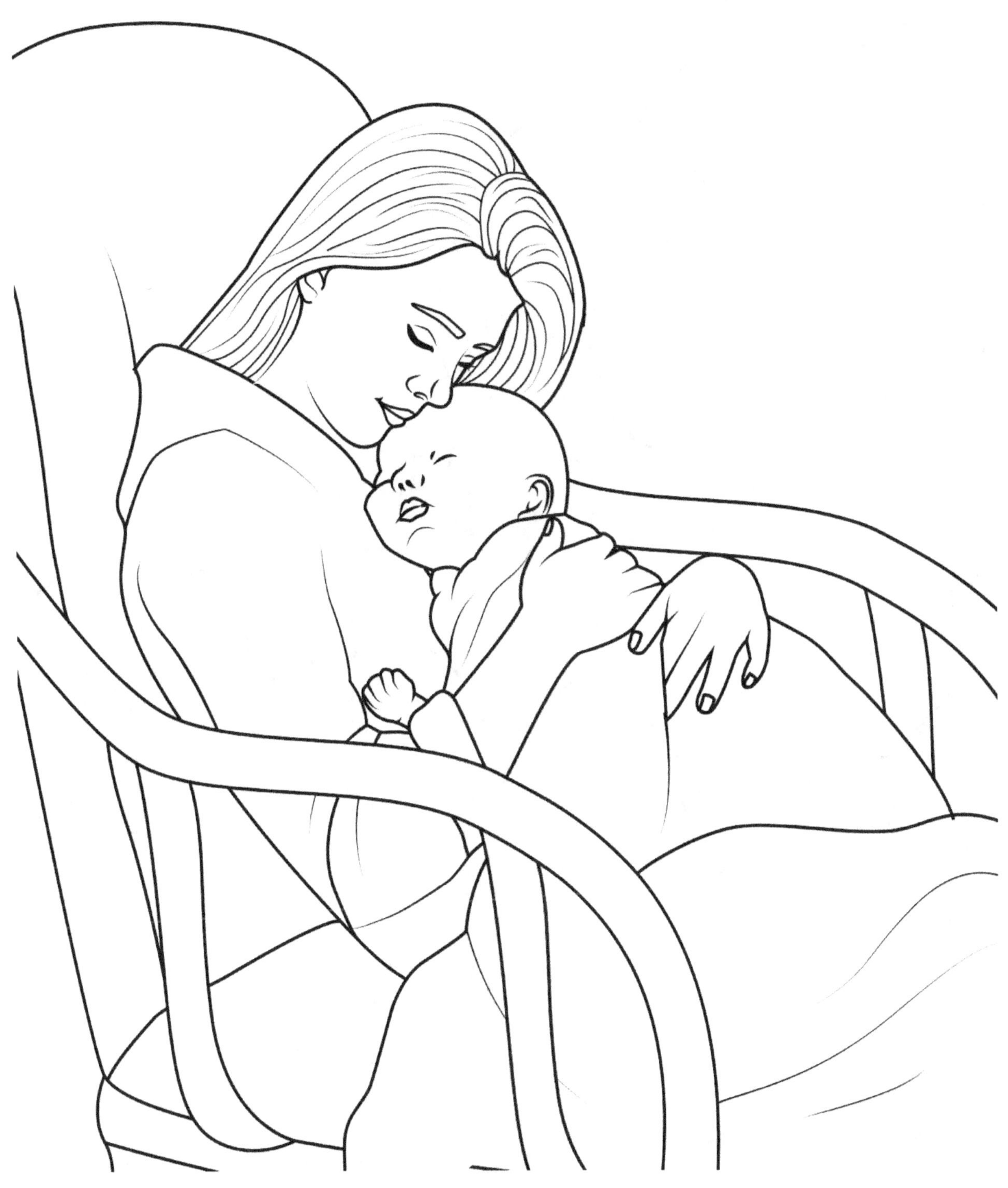

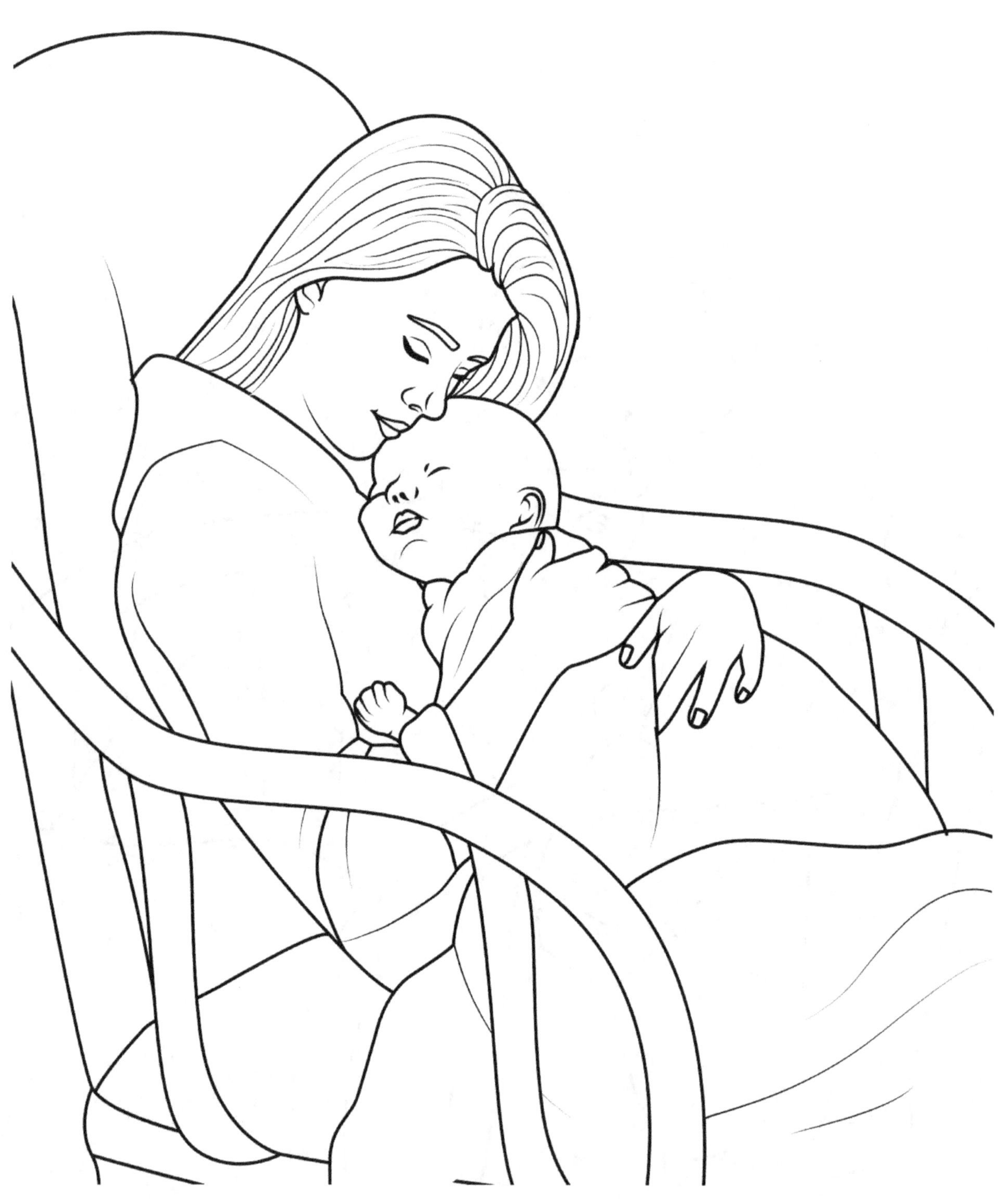

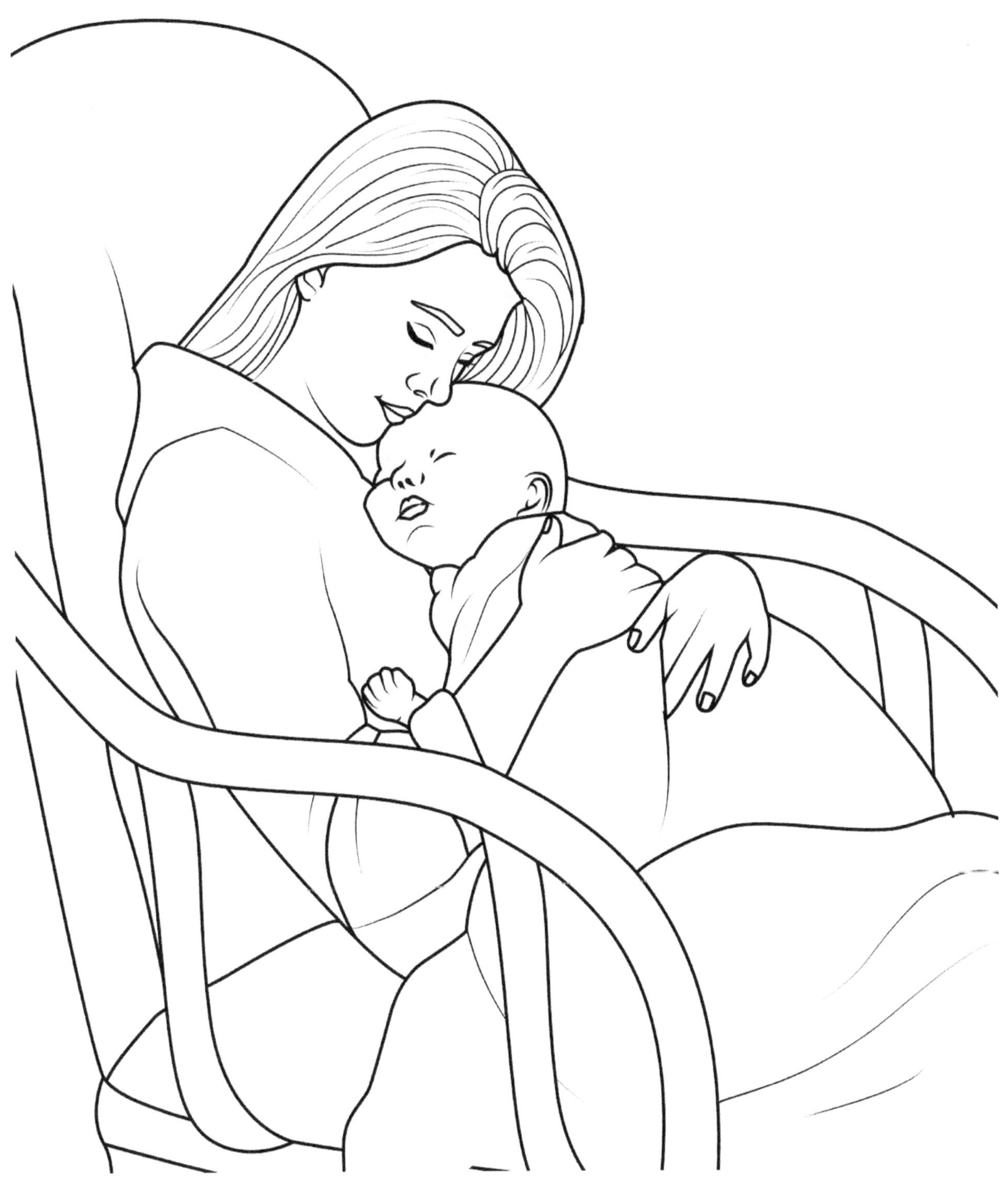

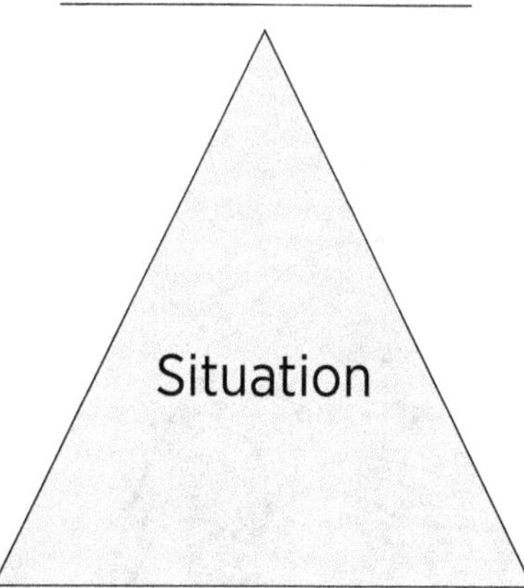

Situation

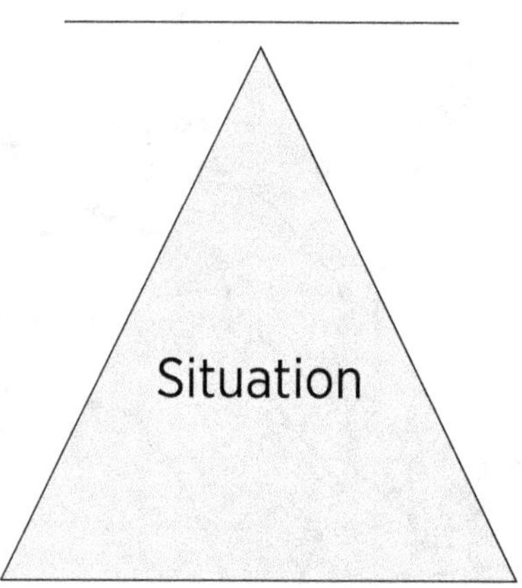

Situation

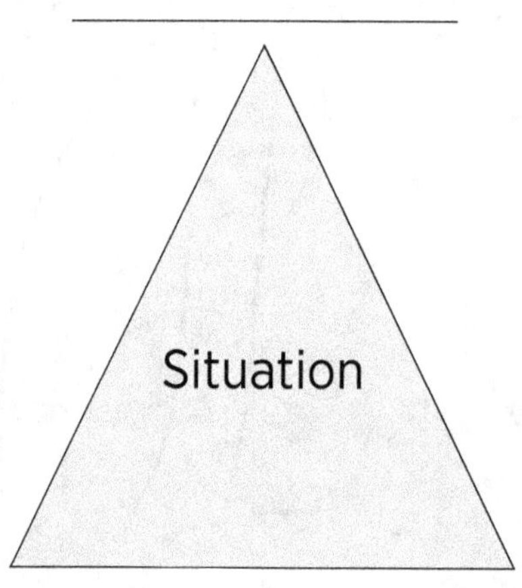

Situation